SIX WEEKS

SIX WEEKS

THE SIX 8110

Caroline Macleod

To order additional copies of this book, contact:
Xlibris
UK TFN: 0800 0148620 (Toll Free inside the UK)
UK Local: 02036 956328 (+44 20 3695 6328 from outside the UK)
www.Xlibrispublishing.co.uk
Orders@Xlibrispublishing.co.uk
824177

CONTENTS

CASSEROLE DISH

HOT SWEETHEART PORK 3
MUSHROOM AND LEEK SOUP 5
MINCED STEW 7
LAMB CHOP 9
TOMATO AND BEEF STEW WITH BREAD 11
TOMATO PASTA 13

DELIGHT DELIVERED

MASH PIE 17
LENTIL SOUP 19
TRIPPY ICE-CREAM 21
SORBET TART' 23

DIP MAGIC

CHICKPEA DIP..27
AVOCADO DIP 29
AUBERGINE DIP 31
CELERY DIP 33
SMOKED SALMON DIP 35

BRIE TISH DIP 37

PARALLEL 40 39

EATING SPANISH... 43

HONORS 45

CASSEROLE DISH

HOT SWEETHEART PORK

One pot cooking at 150 C.

2 Chop

1onion slices

Chilli

Ginger

Soy sauce

Sugar

½ pint gravy

Dry stock.

All in one pot in oven for ¾ HR.

MUSHROOM AND LEEK SOUP

Dry stock

Mushrooms

LEEKS

Milk

Flour

Salt

Rapeseed oil

Put the mushroom and Leek and dry stock in a pan. Add oil. Sweat. Add tablespoon of flour. Stir for a bit. Add milk. Bring to the boil. Stirring. Add salt.

MINCED STEW

Casserole dish filled with mince, mushrooms, onion and soy sauce, stock in gravy and salt. Put in oven 150c for 1 hour. Drain some excess fluid and put mash on the top. Cheese on top. Put in oven for 10-15 minutes.

LAMB CHOP

Leg chop

Soy sauce

White beans tin

Tomatoes chopped tin

Onion

Stock

Gravy

Sugar

Salt

Place in casserole dish in oven at 150c for 2 and a half hours.

TOMATO AND BEEF STEW WITH BREAD

Cook for one and a half hours or two and a half hour at 150c.

Chilli

Ginger

Light Soy sauce

Stock

Salt

Beef

Can of tomato in oil and herbs.

Onion

Sugar

Carrots and potatoes in can.

TOMATO PASTA

Pasta

Cream

Tomatoes with herbs and oil can

Soy sauce light

Cook pasta. Add other things and cook through.

PRAWN COCKTAIL

SQUATTIES AND PRAWNS.

CHEESE SAUCE AND ANY PASSATA TO DIP THEM IN.

DELIGHT DELIVERED

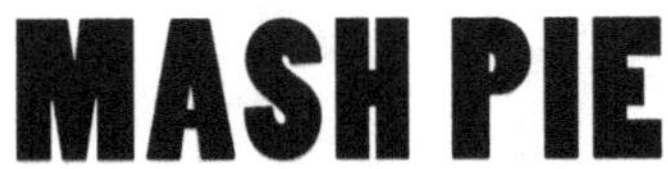

MASH PIE

TIN OF CHOPPED CARROTS.

SMALL ONION FINELY SLICED

STOCK CUBE

MINCE 250G

GRAVY QUART

POTATOES MASHED/SLICES

COOK MEAT CARROTS ONION IN FRYING
PAN LIGHT. STOCK AND QUART ADD.
BUBBLE THROUGH GENTLY. SEASON. INTO
CASSEROLE. MASH ON TOP. OVEN 180C 15
MINUTES. KETCHUP. ORANGE.

LENTIL SOUP

WATER IN PAN. SALT.

ADD RED SPLIT LENTILS. CHOPPED ONION. LEEKS. STOLID. COOK HALF HOUR. NICE STIR.

TRIPPY ICE-CREAM

WHIPPED CREAM.

WHIP EGGS SUGAR AND SIEVE.

ADD DROP OF COINTREAU. WHISKY.

MIX TOGETHER AND FREEZE.

SORBET TART'

Lemon ● grated then cut in half and squeezed into egg and sugar froth.

Add a touch of SALT.

Get some vanilla ice cream.

Mix together.

DIP MAGIC

CHRISTMAS TIME
CRISPS TIME

CHICKPEA DIP

1 can of chickpeas

Soy sauce

Ginger

Garlic

Golden syrup

Salt

Water

Rapeseed oil

Put in a blender.

Dip and enjoy.

AVOCADO DIP

Favourite Spirit

Soured cream

Avocado

Chillies

Put in a blender.

Dip and be merry.

AUBERGINE DIP

Cognac

Roasted Aubergine

Rapeseed oil

Salt

Put in a blender.

Christmas joy.

CELERY DIP

Carrots can of

White wine

Soured cream

Celery hearts in a can

Put in a blender.

Dancer and Prancer Christmas.

SMOKED SALMON DIP

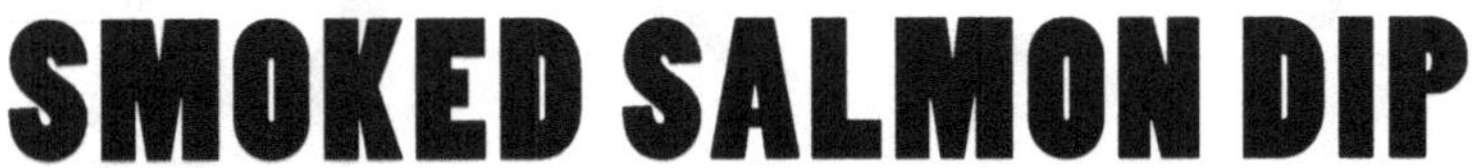

Brandy

Packet of smoked salmon

Mascarpone

Salt and ground pepper

Put in a blender.

Holly and Mistletoe.

Please don't make a rollmops dip. It causes sugar rushes which can make you faint out of conscious.

BRIE TISH DIP

Warm a Brie or Camembert in the oven at 125c with salt and rapeseed oil sprinkled on top. To crisp and bracken the outer edges.

Dip and enjoy.

PARALLEL 40

1. Eat Vegetables when you can.

2. Eating I'd like.

3. Cook. First boil Brussels sprouts in salted water. Then add grated carrots and Mozzarella with chillies to a rapeseed oil and fry. Drain Brussels

sprouts, mash and add to with mentioned ingots.

Eat/drink something sweet like a lemon pancake?

4. Mix self-raising flour and an egg and some cream and add lemon juice. Fry. Serve with some honey.

5. Cook Broccoli well until soft. Put affordable cheese sauce on top. Try serving it with chopped roasted Swede/turnip.

Sorbet for something sweet if you like.

6. Whip up egg whites and add sugar and whip again. Add cream and grated lemon rind and juice. Freeze.

7. LEEKS and white sauce from a packet. Cook Leeks well in salted

water. Eat with Mushrooms and couscous; fry in rapeseed oil until well cooked. Put couscous in a pan and add water to cover. Heat until boiling. Keep adding water.

Chocolate for something sweet. How about Hazelnut meringue with chocolate cream?

8. Make a meringue as usual and put in half an ounce of ground hazelnuts. Bake in 2 cake tins at 125c for 2 hours. For chocolate cream make whipped cream and hot chocolate powder and a little Cassis.

EATING SPANISH

Octopus are intelligent animals that takes food from it's own land. Spanish eat them for this reason so popular. It is a Cult: Fruit Of The Sea.

For the sauce fry and mash potatoes and tomato and add pimento.

Tortilla:/. Onion, potato, egg, chorizo.

Fry onion and potatoes. Pour over beaten egg and add chorizo. Cook further and then grill the top.

Prawn, fry with garlic and butter and Rum.

Lobster, cheese grated and tomato PASSATA with oil and herbs and Vodka.

HONORS

Manner of speaking with food.

Example: In Death you are still living.

Eat to your account.

Wash dishes when applicable.

Hold your own way.

Sleep when you want too.

Wash Par Terre as desired.

Toilet at will.

Mood is Mood.

Eating cures a mood.

Speak at Will.

Someone will hear you.

Good orderly manner.

Discreet fashion.

Pheasants originated in China.

Mildred: 1st Storey: Who gets Murdered?

Ans.: He does. The Little Tin Men.

Nudity; Like I saye, little Robin in the garden.

Happy; like I am.

Glasses; Specs.

It's all love; in love and War.

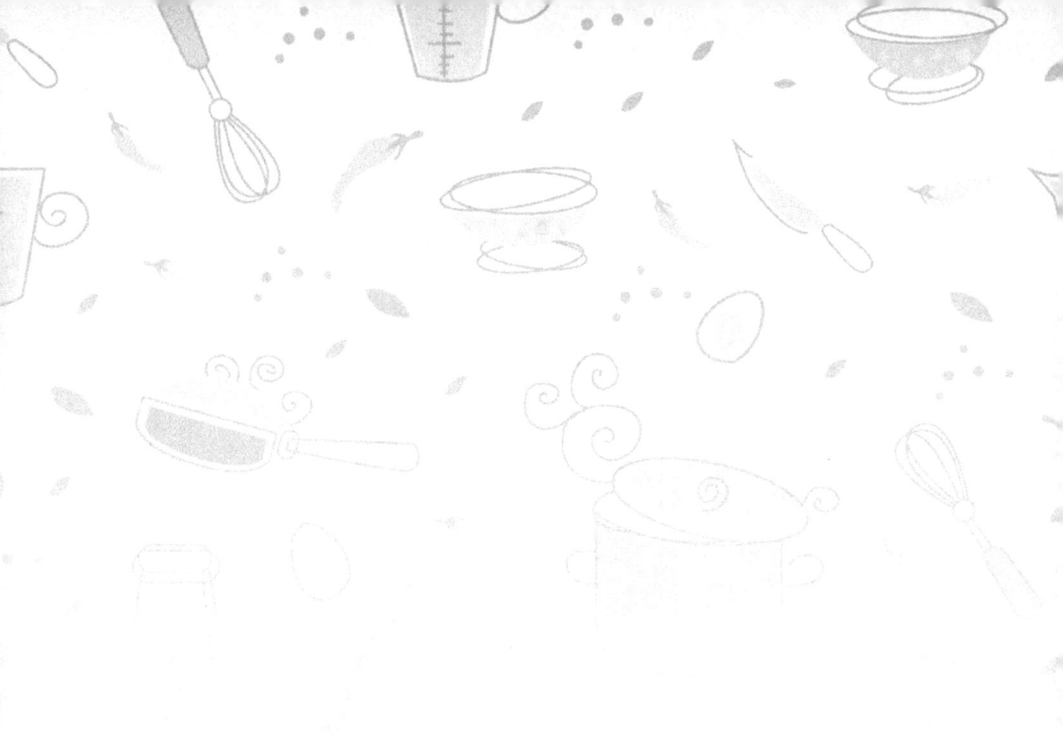

9 781664 114050